FAST FACTS

Indispensable

Guides to

Clinical

Practice

Michael Bailey

Consultant Urologist,
St George's Hospital,
London, UK

Michael Sarosdy

Clinical Professor,
Division of Urology,
University of Texas
Health Science Center,
San Antonio, Texas, USA

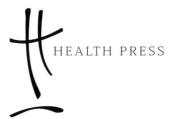

HEALTH PRESS

Oxford

Fast Facts – Bladder Cancer
First published 1999
Reprinted 2000

Text © 2000 Michael Bailey, Michael Sarosdy
© 2000 in this edition Health Press Limited
Elizabeth House, Queen Street, Abingdon, Oxford OX14 3JR, UK

Tel: +44 (0)1235 523233
Fax: +44 (0)1235 523238

Fast Facts is a trade mark of Health Press Limited

A CIP catalogue record for this title is available from the British Library.

ISBN 1-899541-56-X

Bailey, M. (Michael)
Fast Facts – Bladder Cancer/
Michael Bailey, Michael Sarosdy

Illustrated by MeDee Art, London, UK

Printed by Fine Print (Services) Limited, Oxford, UK

Glossary 4

Epidemiology and aetiology 5

Pathology 8

Clinical presentation 14

Investigations 19

Microscopic haematuria 24

Management of superficial disease 28

Management of muscle-invasive disease 35

Management of advanced disease 44

Future trends 49

Key references 52

Index 56

Glossary

Anaplasia: loss of typical cell characteristics or differentiation that can occur, for example, in rapidly growing malignant tumours

BCG: bacillus Calmette-Guérin, a strain of tubercle bacteria that, though it does not cause tuberculosis, can stimulate an immune response

BTA *stat*™ test: bladder tumour antigen test

BTA TRAK™ test: quantifies bladder tumour antigen

CIS: carcinoma *in situ*

CT: computed tomography

Cystectomy: surgical removal of the bladder

Cystoscopy: examination of the bladder using a cystoscope

Dysplasia: abnormal development of tissues, e.g. skin, bone

HPF: high-powered field

IVU: intravenous urogram

MRI: magnetic resonance imaging

NMP-22® test: test for nuclear matrix protein that is secreted by some bladder tumours

Primary CIS: isolated carcinoma *in situ*

RBC: red blood cell

Secondary CIS: carcinoma *in situ* with associated papillary or solid tumours

TCC: transitional cell carcinoma

TNM: tumour–nodes–metastases, a staging system

Urography: radiographical examination of the kidneys using contrast medium

UTI: urinary tract infection

CHAPTER 1
Epidemiology and aetiology

Incidence

The incidence of bladder cancer has risen over the past 20 years. Currently around 54 500 new cases of bladder cancer are diagnosed in the USA each year, and 10 000 cases are diagnosed in the UK annually. Bladder cancer is the fourth most frequently occurring cancer in males in the USA and is the eighth most common cause of mortality. In the UK, it accounts for 5000 deaths per annum.

The incidence of bladder cancer varies among different patient groups. For example, there is a 3:1 male to female ratio, similar to that seen for renal cell carcinoma. The incidence is higher in elderly populations, with a higher percentage of well-differentiated tumours in those who present under the age of 30 years. No evidence exists for a familial or inherited pattern among any patient group. A decreased incidence exists in black people compared with white people and the lifetime risk for developing bladder cancer is:

- 2.8% for white men
- 0.9% for black men
- 1.0% for white women
- 0.6% for black women.

Five-year survival for both black and white people during 1986–92 (60% and 82%, respectively) was significantly improved over the equivalent survival rates during 1974–76 (47% and 74%, respectively; $p < 0.05$).

Aetiology

A number of factors have been implicated in the development of bladder cancer and most relate to environmental carcinogens found in an industrialized society (Table 1.1). Part of the recent decrease in incidence of bladder cancer is probably associated with a decrease in tobacco use, as well as efforts to improve environmental conditions.

Cigarette smoking. Smoking is now recognized as the number one cause of bladder cancer in industrialized countries, with a two- to five-fold increase in the risk of bladder cancer due to smoking. Some 25% of cancers in

TABLE 1.1

Known bladder carcinogens

- 2-naphthylamine
- Benzidine
- 4-aminobiphenyl
- Dichlorobenzidine
- Orthodianisidine
- Orthotolidine
- Phenacitin
- Chlornaphazine
- Cyclophosphamide

TABLE 1.2

Industries in which workers may be exposed to carcinogens

- Chemical dye manufacture
- Rubber manufacture (especially tyres and cables)
- Production of coal gas
- Sewage work
- Manufacture of firelighters
- Pest control
- Textile printing

industrialized countries are due to smoking. Smokers have a higher incidence of tumour recurrences, as well as a higher proportion of tumours of higher stage and grade than do non-smokers. The correlation between smoking and cancer is reportedly higher with bladder cancer than with lung cancer.

Occupational exposure. The highest association of work exposure and bladder cancer is among aniline dye workers who are exposed to aromatic amines, with a relative increased risk ranging from 1.7 to 8.8. Other occupations with increased exposure in the workplace are shown in Table 1.2.

Dietary factors. Caffeine has been implicated in bladder cancer but the relationship has been hard to define due to the widespread use of caffeine, as well as its association with a variety of other known carcinogens, such as smoking. Artificial sweeteners have also been implicated, but the studies undertaken involved extremely high doses and recent efforts to clarify this relationship have failed to do so.

Drugs. Certain drugs have been linked with bladder cancer, including phenacetin (not licensed in the UK), which is especially associated with tumours of the renal pelvis. Cyclophosphamide has also been linked with bladder cancer in both animal and human studies, with patients having a high rate of muscle-invasive tumours and a short time period (6–13 years) between exposure and diagnosis. Prophylactic administration of 2-mercaptoethanesulphonic acid (mesna) may prevent both cyclophosphamide-related cystitis and cancer.

Radiation. Radiotherapy for cervical cancer or for thyroid disease can result in a four-fold and three-fold increase in the risk of bladder cancer, respectively.

Chronic infection/inflammation. Chronic infection or inflammation with indwelling suprapubic catheters in patients with spinal cord injury has been associated with an increased incidence of bladder cancer, especially squamous cell cancer. Schistosomiasis, caused by the organism *Schistosoma haematobium* (Figure 1.1), has been associated with an incidence of bladder cancer as high as 70% in areas of Egypt, where it is the most common cause of bladder cancer.

Chromosomal changes. Increasingly, genetic changes are being linked with bladder cancers. Chief among these are alterations in the tumour suppressor genes *p53* and *Rb* (retinoblastoma gene). Such changes are found more commonly in tumours of high grade and stage.

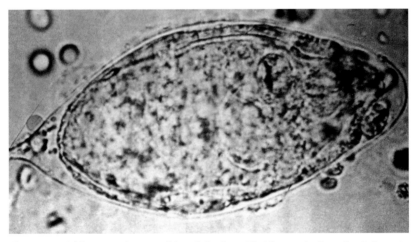

Figure 1.1 *Schistosoma haematobium*: infection with this parasite is endemic in parts of Africa and may cause squamous cell carcinoma of the bladder.

CHAPTER 2

Pathology

Histology

The following histological types of carcinoma occur in the bladder.

Transitional cell cancer (TCC). Derived from the transitional epithelium, TCC accounts for almost 90% of the bladder cancers seen in industrialized countries such as the USA and the UK (Figure 2.1). Most of the discussion on bladder cancer revolves around this type. Such tumours may be papillary and superficial (70–75%) or solid and invasive (20–25%). An additional and important type seen in about 10% is carcinoma *in situ* (CIS), a flat intraepithelial anaplastic carcinoma, often with increased numbers of mitotic structures. Approximately half of the CIS occurs as an isolated lesion (primary CIS), while the remainder occur in association with either papillary or solid tumours (secondary CIS).

Squamous cell carcinoma. Usually an invasive lesion, squamous cell carcinoma has a nodular, infiltrative growth pattern. This comprises about 5–10% of bladder cancers in the US and UK, but up to 70% of bladder cancers in areas where schistosomiasis is endemic, such as Egypt. It is also associated with chronic infection or inflammation, such as with indwelling suprapubic catheters.

Adenocarcinoma is a rare type of bladder carcinoma, accounting for about 2% of bladder cancers. Approximately 30–35% of these are urachal in origin and location, while the remainder are associated with bladder exstrophy or are non-urachal in origin. The urachus is the remnant of the embryonic cavity, the allantois; it usually forms a fibrous cord connecting the bladder to the umbilicus.

Adenocarcinomas are usually solitary, high grade and ulcerative. They are indistinguishable histologically from adenocarcinoma of the colon or rectum, and clinical determination of source of origin is often difficult. Many have a poor prognosis due to advanced stage at the time of diagnosis. Urachal adenocarcinomas, in particular, have a poor prognosis because of

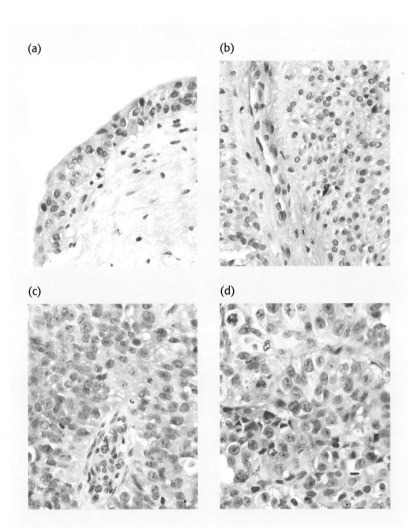

Figure 2.1 Histological sections through the urothelium. Normal urothelium (a) is 5–7 cells thick, and lies between a basement membrane and an intact layer of umbrella cells on the luminal surface. In grade 1 papillary transitional cell carcinoma (TCC; b), urothelial cells have a slightly increased nucleus to cell ratio, and umbrella cells are lost. A fibrovascular stalk is usually prominent. Grade 2 papillary TCC (c) is associated with a large nucleus to cell ratio. There are occasional nucleoli, with some maintenance of cell polarity. With grade 3 TCC (d), a wide range of cell shapes and sizes is seen. The nucleus to cell ratio is very high, mitosis is occasional to frequent, and many multiple nucleoli occur.

the late onset of symptoms due to the minimally functional portion of the bladder in which they arise.

Undifferentiated carcinomas are small cell carcinomas that have a very high nuclear to cytoplasmic ratio, and usually form sheets or nests of cells. They behave like small cell cancer of the lung, and prognosis is poor.

'Field changes' of a probable premalignant nature are often found in association with bladder cancer, and range from atypia to mild or severe dysplasia. The recognition of such changes is important in determining the prognosis of patients relative to the future risk of recurrence or progression. Normal transitional epithelium has a superficial layer of large, flat, umbrella cells, beneath which are three to seven layers of regular cells. These lie above a basement membrane that separates the mucosa from the underlying muscularis. Field changes that may be present include the following.

Atypia indicates that an increased number of cell layers is present, with loss of polarity of a still intact umbrella layer.

Dysplasia. Graded as mild, moderate or severe, dysplasia consists of an increase in the size of nuclei that are basally located and exhibit loss of the usual polarity. The cell layers are not increased in number. Severe dysplasia may be indistinguishable from CIS.

Staging

Tumour–nodes–metastases (TNM) staging is the system most commonly used (Figure 2.2). Prognosis for all stages is highly dependent on accurate clinical staging, as is the selection of adjuvant therapy for superficial disease or CIS.

Grading

A three-grade system of scoring the degree of anaplasia has been adopted by most pathologists (Table 2.1).

Patterns of recurrence and spread

Most superficial Ta and T1 tumours can be completely resected and treated successfully without cystectomy. Approximately 40% of such patients will have no further recurrence after resection of the primary tumour, but initially these cannot be distinguished with certainty from those whose tumours will recur. Also, 20–30% of patients who do experience recurrence

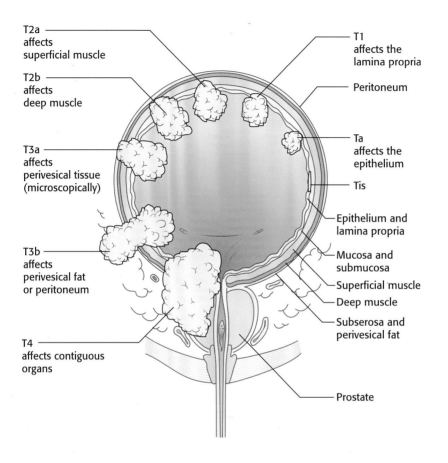

T2a
affects
superficial muscle

T2b
affects
deep muscle

T3a
affects
perivesical tissue
(microscopically)

T3b
affects
perivesical fat
or peritoneum

T4
affects contiguous
organs

T1
affects the
lamina propria

Peritoneum

Ta
affects the
epithelium

Tis

Epithelium and
lamina propria

Mucosa and
submucosa

Superficial muscle

Deep muscle

Subserosa and
perivesical fat

Prostate

Figure 2.2 TNM staging of bladder cancer. It is based on the level of invasion into or through the bladder wall, the involvement of lymph nodes and distant sites of disease.

may suffer progression to a higher stage (see Chapter 6). Consequently, vigilant surveillance is necessary, as is judicious use of intravesical agents to decrease recurrences and progression in high-risk patients (for example, those with large or multiple tumours, high-grade lesions, or superficial tumours with associated CIS or severe dysplasia).

Most recurrences after an initial bladder cancer will be found in the bladder, although 4–10% of patients will develop a tumour in the upper

11

TABLE 2.1
Grading system for anaplasia in bladder cancer

Grade 1: Tumours have the least degree of anaplasia compatible with the diagnosis of cancer

Grade 2: Tumours have a degree of anaplasia between grades 1 and 3

Grade 3: Tumours have the most severe degree of anaplasia

tract and a similar number may develop a tumour in the prostatic urethra. Conversely, 40% of patients who have an initial TCC of the renal pelvis will subsequently develop transitional cell tumours in the bladder.

CIS has a high rate of progression to invasive muscle disease if it is not adequately eradicated with adjuvant therapy or surgical resection. It may also spread to lymph nodes, without first going through a recognized progression to muscle-invasive disease.

Muscle-invasive disease has a high rate of direct spread to regional structures such as pelvic muscles, lymphatic spread to regional lymph nodes, and haematogenous spread to lungs, viscera and bones.

Mortality

Mortality of TCC is directly related to the pathological stage of bladder cancer. For Ta and low-grade T1 tumours, 5-year survival should exceed 95%. For high-grade T1 cancers or CIS, reported 5-year survival without adjuvant therapy may be as low as 50%. If adequate bacillus Calmette-Guérin (BCG) immunotherapy is used, 5-year survival should approach 90–95%. Patients with T2/T3aN0M0 disease have only a 60–70% 5-year survival, despite complete surgical excision. This surprisingly low disease-specific survival is due to the progression of subclinical 'micrometastases', which were present at the time of cystectomy but were not radiologically detectable. Some 80% of these cases develop within 2 years of cystectomy, with the remainder presenting between years 2 and 4.

Patients with T4 (N+ or M+) disease have a 5-year survival of only 10–20%. Patients with adenocarcinoma or squamous carcinoma have reasonably good prognosis following complete surgical excision unless nodal disease is found. Those with nodal disease or in whom distant metastases are present at diagnosis have a uniformly poor outcome.

CHAPTER 3
Clinical presentation

The classical presenting symptom of a patient with a bladder tumour is painless haematuria. This symptom is usually taken seriously by the patient and their primary care physician, and appropriate action initiated. However, other presentations are not uncommon (Table 3.1) and are sometimes unrecognized as an indication of serious underlying pathology.

TABLE 3.1
Presenting symptoms

Symptom	Description
Painless haematuria	Visible passage of blood in urine, without associated pain, frequency or dysuria. Up to 30% of patients will have urinary tract malignancy
Microscopic haematuria	Presence of red blood cells in the urine of insufficient quantity to be visible to the naked eye, without urological symptoms. About 10% of these patients will have malignant disease
Irritative symptoms	Dysuria, frequency, suprapubic pain with a full bladder. Some 25% of patients with bladder tumours will have one or more of these symptoms
Recurrent urinary tract infection	In older (i.e. 50+ years) patients with recurrent bacterial cystitis, the possibility of an underlying tumour should be considered
Systemic symptoms	Loin pain, weight loss, malaise, anorexia, bone pain, pathological fracture, cough

Painless haematuria

Painless haematuria may occur at the beginning, the end or throughout the stream of urine. It may be profuse, so that the patient complains of passing pure blood and the urine may contain clots, or there may be only a slight pink discoloration of the urine. If there have been clots in the bladder for some time, they may impart a rusty colour to the urine. Any patient complaining of these symptoms should be referred to a urologist immediately. Patients will sometimes ignore a single episode of bleeding and delay seeking advice until the bleeding recurs. This can lead to significant delay in diagnosis and treatment, with the result that treatment may be more difficult and the chance of cure reduced. Haematuria, either painless or microscopic, is the sole presenting symptom in 80% of patients with carcinoma of the bladder.

Asymptomatic microscopic haematuria

As screening programmes and medical examinations for insurance purposes become more widespread, the finding of microscopic (dipstick) haematuria is increasing. Because this is now such a common finding, microscopic haematuria is covered separately in Chapter 5. Microscopic haematuria must be regarded as part of the spectrum of painless haematuria and should always be investigated.

Irritative symptoms

Dysuria, increased frequency and urgency are usually due to urinary tract infection (UTI). If infection is absent or symptoms persist after treating the infection, however, the possibility of an underlying bladder carcinoma must be considered. Suprapubic pain when the bladder is full can also be due to carcinoma of the bladder. These irritative symptoms are especially common in patients with CIS. Irritative symptoms are very common and are usually not associated with serious disease, so it is very easy for patients and their primary care physicians to dismiss them. Urinalysis in patients with irritative symptoms due to CIS or invasive cancer will usually indicate red or white blood cells, and if urine cytology is requested, may show malignant cells. Persistent symptoms in the absence of documented UTI should result in referral to a urologist. Up to 20% of patients with bladder cancer will *not* have haematuria at the time of presentation.

Recurrent urinary traction infections

Recurrent infections are sometimes due to the presence of a bladder tumour. A single infection in a male, or two or more infections in a female should be investigated. The likelihood of a malignant aetiology in patients under 50 years of age is, however, very small.

Systemic symptoms

Patients will sometimes present with systemic systems due to advanced carcinoma of the bladder. Loin pain can be due to ureteric obstruction by an invasive bladder tumour (Figure 3.1). The pain is usually a dull ache in the renal angle, and may or may not coincide with other symptoms such as haematuria. Occasionally, infection will occur in such a situation, giving rise to severe symptoms of pyelonephritis. Coughing or chest pain may be due to pulmonary metastases (Figure 3.2); the cough in usually non-productive. Pleuritic chest pain may also occur. Anorexia, nausea, weight loss and malaise may result from renal failure due to bilateral ureteric obstruction, or from the systemic effects of the tumour itself. Bone pain or pathological fractures may result from skeletal metastases; the pain is unrelieved by rest and can be very severe (Figure 3.3). Anaemia and hypercalcaemia may occur as metabolic complications of advanced disease.

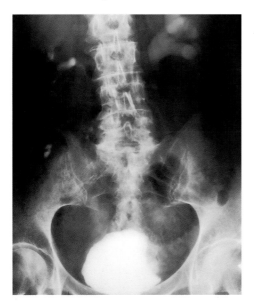

Figure 3.1 Intravenous urogram showing ureteric obstruction by a bladder tumour, which is usually a sign of an invasive tumour.

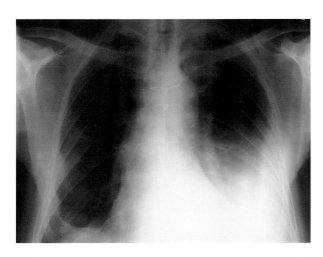

Figure 3.2 Chest radiograph showing multiple pulmonary metastases.

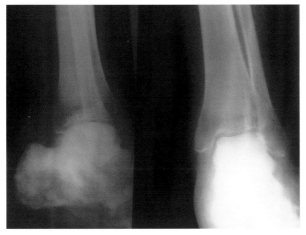

Figure 3.3 Bone destruction by secondary deposits from an invasive bladder tumour. When present in a weight-bearing bone, pathological fracture may occur.

Delay in diagnosis

Although the evidence that delay in diagnosis affects prognosis is far from conclusive, it seems desirable to ensure prompt diagnosis and treatment for patients with bladder cancer. Delays may occur for a variety of reasons.

- Patient delay: anxiety about the cause of the symptoms, fear of primary care physician or hospitals, or ignorance about the significance of symptoms.
- Delay in referral from the primary care physician to a specialist: ignorance of the significance of the symptoms, limited access to specialist healthcare (waiting times for clinic appointments).

- Delay in specialist reaching a diagnosis: waiting times for investigations, waiting time to attend follow-up clinics for results, waiting list delays for cystoscopy.

The sum of these factors means that the average time from the patient first noticing a symptom to the time of treatment of the bladder tumour varies in different studies from 85 days to as long as 6 months.

In an attempt to streamline diagnosis and treatment of patients with symptoms suggestive of bladder cancer, many hospitals now offer a haematuria service at which patients can be seen within a week of referral. The clinic should be able to perform urine cytology and dipstick analysis for blood and leucocytes, intravenous urography and flexible cystoscopy on the same day. This allows a diagnosis to be made and treatment planned expeditiously.

CHAPTER 4

Investigations

History and examination

A thorough history should be obtained from all patients presenting with symptoms. This should include history of smoking, possible carcinogen exposure in the workplace, history of previous bladder tumour resection and history of any change in bowel habits or stool characteristics. Direct questioning may reveal a history of mild intermittent gross haematuria for 6–12 months prior to actual presentation.

Physical examination is usually unremarkable in cases of superficial bladder cancer unless acute urinary retention is present with bladder distension. In men, a careful rectal examination is important to exclude prostatic disease such as cancer or benign enlargement, both of which may be associated with many of the symptoms of bladder cancer, and to rule out gross extension of bladder cancer. A careful pelvic examination is equally important in women. Attention should be paid to a thorough nodal examination, including supraclavicular lymph nodes.

Urinalysis should include both dipstick and microscopic analysis to rule out infection and assess the level of microscopic blood present if the urine is grossly free of blood. Cytology should not be obtained in the initial evaluation of haematuria, as the majority of haematuria cases are not due to malignant causes. Instead, it should be reserved for cases in which the evaluation is otherwise negative. Similarly, new diagnostic tests recently introduced for bladder cancer (BTA *stat*™, Bard; NMP-22®, Matritech) should not be performed in the initial evaluation of haematuria, but reserved for use in patients after the diagnosis of bladder cancer.

Radiographic studies should include an intravenous urogram (IVU) after appropriate preparation of the patient. If superficial cancer is subsequently discovered, seen as a smooth or irregular filling defect displacing contrast in the bladder (Figure 4.1), additional studies are not warranted. However, if muscle-invasive disease is found, pelvic and possibly abdominal computed

19

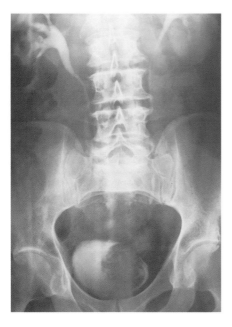

Figure 4.1 Intravenous urogram showing large filling defect. This patient had ignored her haematuria for 12 months and although the tumour was large, it was not invasive.

tomography (CT) should be obtained to assess pelvic and retroperitoneal lymph nodes, adjacent organs and the liver. Ultrasonography of the kidneys may be obtained in cases of contrast allergy or uraemia (to avoid potential renal failure). Ultrasonography and magnetic resonance imaging (MRI) of the bladder or the tumour do not provide clinically useful information and are not warranted. MRI of the abdomen and pelvis does not provide any additional information over CT scanning and, due to its higher cost, is not justified.

Cystoscopy is required to determine the presence or absence of small tumours that may not be seen in the bladder views of the IVU. It may usually be accomplished under local anaesthetic using a flexible cystoscope (Figure 4.2). If a bladder tumour is obvious on the IVU, then cystoscopy under local anaesthetic may be omitted. Instead, the patient may be taken directly to the operating suite for rigid endoscopy under anaesthesia, with simultaneous resection or biopsy of the tumour.

Cytological examination of exfoliated cells should be obtained in cases of high-grade tumour after resection and after any haematuria has cleared. A bladder wash for cytology should also be obtained at the time of cystoscopy

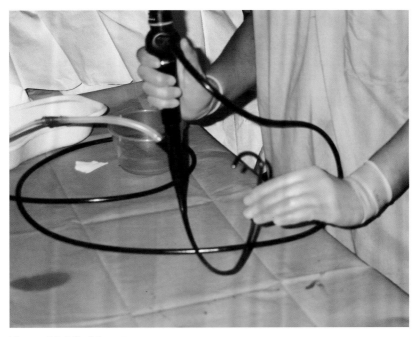

Figure 4.2 A flexible cystoscope.

if areas compatible with CIS or ulcers are seen instead of obvious tumour. Cytology may be helpful in following such patients for future recurrence, as well as ensuring that all disease present at initial diagnosis has been diagnosed and treated adequately. Cytology is relatively insensitive in low-grade disease and is therefore not warranted.

Pathological interpretation of both histology and cytology specimens is critical. Recent reports indicate at least a 30% rate of discordance among pathologists, including many who specialize in uropathology. Because many treatment and prognostic decisions are based upon fine distinctions between grade (3 versus 1 or 2), invasion (T1 versus T2) and field changes (CIS versus mild or moderate dysplasia), it is important that both understaging and overstaging of bladder cancers be minimized. Second-opinion pathology should be routine if the 'pathologist of the day' sees only an occasional case of bladder cancer.

Transurethral resection of the tumour(s) is the mainstay of both diagnosis and initial management. If limited papillary disease is present, as is most often the case, no additional therapy may be required other than regular cystoscopic surveillance. Complete resection may be possible if the tumour is small, solid and muscle invasive (Figure 4.3). However, extensive resections of large, invasive tumours may serve no useful purpose because cystectomy may be needed shortly. In addition, the risk of postoperative bleeding and clot retention is increased. Deep biopsy at the juncture of the tumour and the muscular wall may be sufficient to confirm the diagnosis of muscle involvement.

Biopsy. Mucosal biopsies should be performed in selected cases to rule out or diagnose associated field changes (Figure 4.4). Small, obviously low-grade papillary and superficial tumours, and large, obviously muscle-invasive tumours do not warrant such biopsies. Biopsies should be performed under the following circumstances:
- cases of multiple papillary tumours
- tumours that appear more solid but are resectable
- bladders with erythematous areas that may represent CIS.

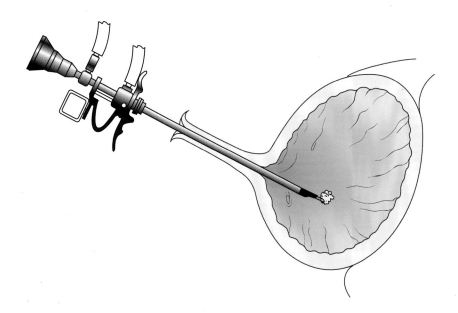

Figure 4.3 Transurethral resection of a small, solid and muscle-invasive tumour.

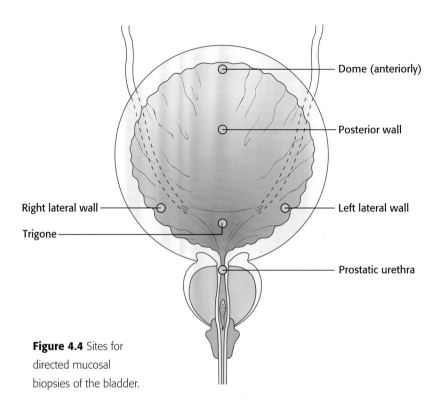

Dome (anteriorly)

Posterior wall

Right lateral wall

Left lateral wall

Trigone

Prostatic urethra

Figure 4.4 Sites for directed mucosal biopsies of the bladder.

Biopsies might also be obtained circumferentially around small, solid, invasive-appearing tumours away from the bladder base or bladder neck in selected cases where partial cystectomy might be considered for definitive therapy.

CHAPTER 5

Microscopic haematuria

Asymptomatic microscopic haematuria may be caused by any of the conditions causing frank painless haematuria, and must be appropriately investigated.

Excretion of red blood cells

Excretion of red blood cells (RBCs) at a rate of 0–1 million per 24 hours is considered normal. If urine is centrifuged and the deposit examined using a high power microscope, this number of red cells would equate to 3–5 RBCs per high-powered field (HPF). Thus the finding of red cells in numbers greater than this may be considered abnormal. It has been suggested that the finding of 5 RBCs/HPF represents the threshold for instigating investigation in asymptomatic individuals.

Collection of urine samples

In order to avoid unnecessary investigation, it is important to collect urine samples in a way that will avoid contamination:

- withdraw the foreskin and clean the glans
- avoid taking samples when the individual is menstruating
- do not take samples after vigorous exercise
- always use freshly voided samples.

False-negative reactions occur with high vitamin C levels or contamination with formalin.

Reagent testing

Dipsticks are widely used as an economical and simple screening test to look for the presence of blood, haemoglobin, protein, nitrites, glucose and leucocytes in urine samples (Figure 5.1). The reaction used to detect RBCs or haemoglobin is peroxidase based and the sensitivity of commercial reagent strips is equivalent to 2–5 RBCs/HPF. As dipsticks may be more sensitive to blood in the urine and give a positive result at a lower threshold than that at which further investigation is warranted (i.e. 5 RBCs/HPF), positive dipstick results for haematuria should be confirmed by microscopic urinalysis with

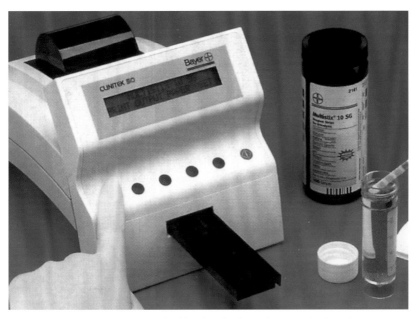

Figure 5.1 A reagent strip to test for blood and other substances in the urine.

the threshold for evaluation set at 5 or more RBCs/HPF. This procedure will decrease the number of investigations following false-positive dipstick results.

Haematuria, whether macroscopic or microscopic, can be intermittent even when there is a urological malignancy, so repeat testing to confirm the finding is not helpful in defining a high-risk group. Age is a significant factor for haematuria. In all reported studies, the number of patients under 40 years of age who were found to have a serious cause for haematuria was very small. Patients in this age group with haematuria and proteinuria should be referred to a nephrologist. It follows, therefore, that if the test has been correctly performed and false-positives excluded, anyone over 40 years of age with haematuria detected by a dipstick should be investigated. Results indicate that 2–5% of patients over 40 years with a positive dipstick test will be found to have a bladder tumour, another 5–10% will have significant pathology such as stone disease, prostate cancer or renal cancer, but the majority will have no detectable cause. In the group with no abnormality detected, there is no increased risk of developing urological disease in the future.

Diagnostic workup

Patients with asymptomatic microscopic haematuria should have a full workup as for frank haematuria. Ultrasound of the renal tract together with a standard radiograph can be substituted for an IVU, but small TCC of the upper tract may be missed. If negative results are found with one imaging modality, then the other modality should be requested.

The results of investigations in patients with haematuria are shown in Table 5.1. If proteinuria is found in association with haematuria, a nephrological cause should be sought. Phase contrast microscopy of the urine may identify dysmorphic or crenelated RBCs characteristic of renal disease. Other population-based studies on the use of microscopic haematuria in diagnosis have shown a low detection rate of bladder

TABLE 5.1

Results of investigations in patients with haematuria*

Diagnosis	Presentation			
	MH	ASM	SM	Total (%)
No urological abnormality	60	52	44	156 (39)
Urinary tract infection	45	5	39	89 (22)
Benign prostatic hyperplasia	44	7	6	57 (14)
Bladder tumour	26	3	2	31 (8)
Stone disease	10	8	2	20 (5)
Renal carcinoma	6	0	0	6 (1.5)
Carcinoma of the prostate	2	3	1	6 (1.5)
Urethral stricture	2	2	1	5 (1.3)
Other (benign)	18	4	2	24 (6)

ASM = asymptomatic microscopic haematuria
MH = macroscopic haematuria
SM = symptomatic microscopic haematuria

*Data from Lynch et al., 1994

carcinoma ranging from 2 to 22%. In one such study of 2700 subjects aged between 35 and 55 years, 13% had one or more RBCs detected in a spun deposit of urine, but only 2% of this group had serious urological disease.

Significance of a negative diagnostic workup

Follow-up studies have been undertaken to quantify the risk of missing a lesion on the standard workup for haematuria. In a study involving 155 patients, no significant pathology was found over a 20-year period. There is therefore no need to retest patients who have been thoroughly evaluated with negative results. It must be stressed that this does not mean the individual concerned can ignore symptoms of urinary tract disease in the future – new pathology can of course develop, and macroscopic haematuria would require re-investigation.

CHAPTER 6
Management of superficial disease

Prognostic factors

Following transurethral resection of the initial tumour and directed biopsies of normal-appearing mucosa, patients with non-invasive, superficial tumours (Ta or T1) may be stratified according to a number of prognostic factors. Table 6.1 shows the grouping of those factors into favourable and unfavourable initial tumour characteristics.

Histological grade and stage. These are the single most useful prognostic factors to date. In the absence of adjuvant therapy after surgery, recurrent tumours will only be seen in up to 50% of patients with grade 1 tumours,

TABLE 6.1

Practical classification of superficial bladder cancers

By superficial tumour characteristics

Favourable	Unfavourable
Single tumour	Multiple tumours
Stage Ta	Stage T1
Low grade	High grade
No field changes	Atypia or dysplasia
Diploid	Aneuploid
Negative cytology	Positive cytology

By characteristics and recurrence history

Nuisance	Favourable characteristics, single occurrence or infrequent recurrences
Troublesome	Favourable characteristics but frequent recurrences
Dangerous	Unfavourable characteristics, any occurrence or recurrences

but in the majority of those with grade 3 tumours. Progression to muscle-invasive disease is rare with grade 1, but may be seen in 11% of grade 2 tumours and in 30–80% of grade 3 tumours. Similarly, for patients with an initial Ta tumour, only 4% will ever progress to T2 or greater, while such progression will be seen in 30% of those with T1, 50% of those with CIS, and up to 80% of those with T1 tumour associated with CIS.

Single versus multiple tumours. The next strongest indicator of prognosis is multiplicity of tumours. A statistically higher percentage of patients with three or more tumours at initial presentation will develop recurrent tumours compared with those who have only one or two tumours at initial presentation.

Atypia, dysplasia and CIS. Mucosal or field changes of atypia, dysplasia and CIS found on random or directed biopsies are ominous indicators of outcome. Progression to muscle invasion is seen in only 7% of those who have a papillary tumour associated with normal mucosa, but in 36% if atypia is present, and in up to 80% if CIS is present.

Prognostic groups
Patients can be stratified into low-, intermediate- and high-risk groups; future therapy, as well as surveillance, may be tailored to this.

Low-risk, nuisance tumours. Patients with a solitary, low-grade Ta lesion are at low risk for recurrence or progression. No adjuvant therapy need be given, as the cost and inconvenience of such therapy cannot be justified. Furthermore, recent experience suggests that if the first surveillance cystoscopy is negative, the interval between surveillance cystoscopies may be increased significantly. Patients who do develop a recurrence of similar stage and grade have been shown to benefit from intravesical chemotherapy.

Intermediate-risk, bothersome tumours. Patients with multiple, low-grade Ta tumours are at intermediate risk of recurrence or progression, particularly if atypia or dysplasia is also present. Similarly, patients with frequent recurrences of low-grade Ta tumours require surgical resection for each recurrence; this is 'bothersome', though not threatening to life or bladder preservation. These patients should be treated initially with intravesical chemotherapy. Intravesical BCG immunotherapy is sometimes used at the outset, but in the majority of cases, it is reserved for treatment failure following chemotherapy.

High-risk, dangerous tumours. Patients who present with CIS or high-grade, high-stage, papillary tumours with or without CIS are at high to very high risk for recurrence and progression. Initial diagnosis should be followed by the administration of intravesical BCG immunotherapy. Recurrence or persistence of disease after one course of BCG places the patient at a greater likelihood of failure, but a second course will effect a response in approximately two-thirds of such patients. Thus, the risk of delaying cystectomy for a second course of therapy is considered reasonable by most urologists.

Intravesical therapy

Anticancer drugs have been used intravesically (Figure 6.1) for bladder cancer for approximately 30 years, with most data demonstrating a modest beneficial effect in prevention of recurrence but not in prevention of progression in stage. Commonly used agents with demonstrated activity include thiotepa, doxorubicin, epirubicin and mitomycin C.

Chemotherapy. The three uses of intravesical chemotherapy are adjunctive, therapeutic and prophylactic. Most therapeutic and prophylactic protocols or regimens are based upon empirical usage and not pharmacological or pharmacokinetic data. However, single-dose, post-therapy, adjunctive use appears to be of value, as do repetitive weekly courses for the prevention of recurrences, particularly among those with low-grade, low-stage tumours. While chemotherapeutic drugs have demonstrated limited therapeutic value in eradicating existing disease, such as residual tumours or CIS, most comparative clinical trials have found BCG immunotherapy to be significantly superior.

Immunotherapy. Intravesical immunotherapy with BCG was first reported to be effective in decreasing papillary tumour recurrence by Morales *et al.* in 1976. Since then, it has been shown to be the most effective agent for

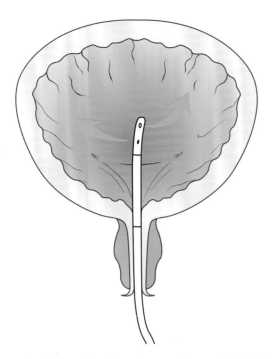

Figure 6.1 Intravesical therapy. The chemotherapeutic agent is instilled into the bladder using a disposable catheter and urethral anaesthesia. The patient is asked to retain the solution for a minimum of an hour, and then expel it by voiding normally. The patient may be asked to move around in order to coat the lining of the bladder with the cytotoxic solution.

prevention of recurrence and has also been shown to prevent tumour progression. BCG immunotherapy is also highly effective in CIS, resulting in complete remission of existing disease in up to 75–80% of those treated with repeated courses. BCG does have increased toxicity over intravesical chemotherapy (Table 6.2). This may be substantial in patients who receive maintenance courses consisting of three consecutive weekly doses every 6 months for up to 3 years after initial induction therapy. For this reason, BCG immunotherapy is usually used initially only in those with high-risk disease, and as a second-line drug for those with lower risk disease but continued recurrences after adequate intravesical chemotherapy. Some of the side-effects of BCG may be prevented or decreased in severity through the prophylactic use of isoniazid for 3 days in conjunction with each intravesical

TABLE 6.2

Complications of BCG immunotherapy in 2602 patients*

Complication	Number (%)
Fever	75 (2.9)
Granulomatous prostatitis	23 (0.9)
Pneumonitis/hepatitis	18 (0.7)
Arthralgia	12 (0.5)
Haematuria	24 (0.9)
Rash	8 (0.3)
Ureteral obstruction	8 (0.3)
Epididymitis	10 (0.4)
Contracted bladder	6 (0.2)
Renal abscess	2 (0.1)
Sepsis	10 (0.4)
Cytopenia	2 (0.1)

*Data from Lamm, 1992

treatment, but this is not yet standard practice. Deaths directly attributable to BCG have occurred, so its use should be restricted to urologists who have developed experience with both its administration and management of its side-effects.

Given the success of BCG immunotherapy, several other immunotherapeutic agents have been investigated. The two with the largest clinical experience are recombinant alpha-2b interferon (Intron A®, Schering-Plough Ltd) and bropirimine. Glashan (1990) reported complete response in 45% of patients with CIS with Intron A, 100 mega units intravesically, delivered at weekly intervals for 12 weeks. Bropirimine is an orally administered interferon inducer and stimulator of other aspects of both cellular and humoral immunity. It has been shown to clear CIS in 50–62% of patients. Both Intron A and bropirimine are able to clear CIS in some patients who had failed previous BCG immunotherapy. Clinical studies of these and other agents are continuing.

Surveillance for recurrence

Surveillance and early detection are necessary. Prior to widespread use of BCG, patients with high-risk disease generally underwent cystectomy and were at risk only of upper tract recurrence (about 4–5%) or urethral recurrence (about 10%) if urethrectomy had not been performed. With the successful treatment of bladder tumours and CIS with BCG, additional bladder recurrences and higher percentages of patients with upper tract recurrence or progression have been reported. While intravesically administered drugs cannot reach the upper tracts without difficult manoeuvres, bropirimine has been reported to eradicate upper tract CIS in 50% of patients. Also, newer technology in the form of small, flexible ureteroscopes allows some small papillary tumours of the upper urinary tract to be resected or laser fulgurated, thus treating the tumour without the need for nephro-ureterectomy.

Cystoscopy. Routine surveillance for superficial bladder tumours has generally consisted of quarterly cystoscopy for 2 years after an initial tumour, semi-annual cystoscopy for an additional 2 years, and annual cystoscopy thereafter if recurrent tumours are never found, as late recurrence can occur. Lifelong surveillance is recommended. If recurrence is detected, the patient starts this schedule again from the beginning. As mentioned previously, it has recently been determined that patients with a single, low-grade Ta tumour and a negative 'first-check cystoscopy' can probably benefit from an immediate increase to a 1-year interval between cystoscopies, as most recurrences in such patients will appear at the first surveillance cystoscopy. In the UK, it is considered safer to discharge patients with low-grade tumours after 10 years of clear cystoscopies. The patient must be told, however, that any episodes of haematuria would require re-investigation.

Cytology. For those patients with high-grade tumours, either papillary or CIS, voided or bladder wash cytology may be helpful as an adjunct to cystoscopy, especially for CIS. However, the yield for cytology is low for low-grade 1 or 2 tumours. For those in whom cytology is important, the test is usually performed at the time of cystoscopy, often with a saline wash of the bladder because the sensitivity is higher than with a voided specimen. Results are not available until several days later, and some expertise is required to perform and interpret the test.

Tumour markers. Several diagnostic tests have been studied recently. One, the BTA *stat* test, has been shown to be approximately twice as sensitive as cytology and is particularly effective for detecting the low- and intermediate-grade tumours that cytology misses. It takes only minutes to carry out and can be performed at the time of cystoscopy. The BTA *stat* test has been available for 1–2 years in the US and Europe, and reports by multiple investigators indicate that it may have a more useful role than cytology, at least in patients for whom cytology would otherwise be indicated. In the UK, surveillance cystoscopy is usually performed in the out-patient setting using a flexible (diagnostic only) scope. One study showed that if patients with a positive BTA *stat* test skipped the flexible cystoscopy and were taken directly to anaesthesia and rigid cystoscopy for possible resection, the cost savings were substantial, even allowing for a few with 'false-negative' rigid cystoscopy results. Trials are planned to determine whether the use of the BTA *stat* test can reduce the use of cystoscopy.

The BTA *stat* test is a second-generation diagnostic test that is performed on unmodified (unbuffered) urine. The method is similar to that of a pregnancy test and the results are available in 5 minutes. The BTA *stat* test detects a different protein from that detected by the original BTA test, and the newer test has a higher sensitivity with specificity similar to that of the original test. A quantitative test, called BTA TRAK™ (Bard), which measures the same protein as that detected by the BTA *stat* test, has also been developed. The level of tumour-associated protein measured by this system appears to correlate directly with increasing stage and grade of tumour. This test may, therefore, allow serial follow up of patients and indicate response to therapy and prognosis for recurring disease.

A similar test that measures a nuclear matrix protein secreted by some bladder tumours has also been developed, and is called the NMP-22 assay. Its prognostic value for eventual tumour recurrence has been evaluated, but to date its value in diagnostic monitoring has not been assessed. Additionally, a number of molecular markers are being studied for prediction of outcome. These markers include *p53* and *Rb*-1 tumour suppressor genes.

CHAPTER 7
Management of muscle-invasive disease

Muscle invasion indicates a poor prognosis in bladder cancer, with overall survival rates of around 50% at 5 years. Radical treatment is necessary if the patient is to be offered a chance of cure. There are two mainstays of treatment – surgical removal of the bladder (cystectomy) or radiotherapy – that can be used alone or in various combinations.

Staging of invasive disease

Prior to deciding on treatment for an individual, as much information as possible about the extent of the disease must be obtained. In patients with T2/T3N0M0 disease, treatment should be offered with curative intent. If the tumour is T2/T3N1M0, cure is unlikely, and with N2 or M1 disease, only palliation can be achieved. Some patients will have T4 tumours because of prostatic involvement, and if N0/M0 may still be cured. A number of investigations can be carried out to identify the stage and grade of the tumour.

Cystoscopy and biopsy with bimanual examination. During cystoscopy in a patient with suspected invasive disease, biopsies should be taken with a resectoscope sufficiently deep to include muscle, in order to allow accurate histological staging and grading of the tumour. At the end of the cystoscopic procedure, with the bladder empty and the patient relaxed, the bladder is palpated bimanually with a finger in the rectum (or vagina in women) and suprapubic pressure applied with the other hand. Clinical staging can thus be established. The presence of a palpable thickening or mass in the bladder wall suggests invasive disease.

CT scanning. This is performed using intravenous, oral and rectal contrast to establish the degree of invasion of the tumour into the bladder and perivesical tissues, as well as to identify lymphadenopathy, ureteric obstruction, or liver or pulmonary metastases. This procedure is usually accurate in identifying extravesical extension of the tumour, but sometimes scarring from previous transurethral resections of the tumour may cause problems with diagnosis (Figure 7.1).

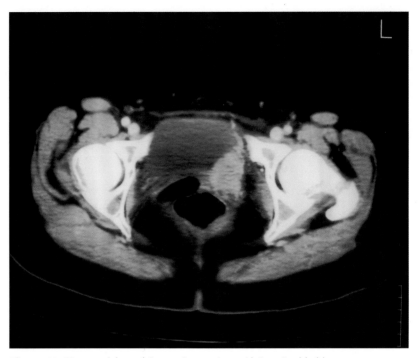

Figure 7.1 CT scan of the pelvic area in a patient with invasive bladder cancer, indicating penetration of the tumour into the perivesical fat.

MRI. This technique, particularly using an endorectal coil, may provide better images of the pelvic organs and allow more accurate assessment of the extent of invasion by the tumour than CT scanning (Figure 7.2).

Chest X-ray. If CT scanning of the chest has not been performed, a chest radiograph is needed to exclude pulmonary metastases, ideally using whole lung tomography.

Bone scanning. Whilst not a routine part of the staging investigation, a bone scan should be obtained if there are any symptoms that might suggest metastasis to bone.

Treatment options

A number of treatment options exists for muscle-invasive bladder cancer (Table 7.1).

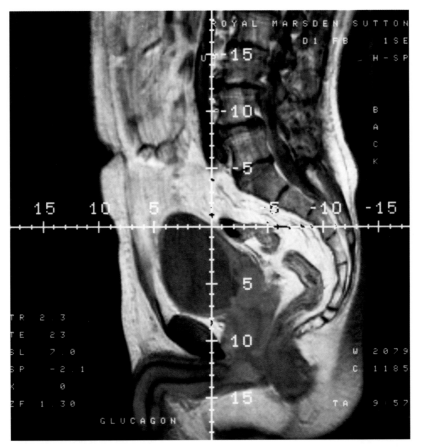

Figure 7.2 MRI scan of the pelvis in a patient with invasive bladder cancer.

TABLE 7.1

Treatment options for muscle-invasive bladder cancer

- Radiotherapy
- Radical surgery:
    - cystectomy with ileal conduit urinary diversion
    - cystectomy with orthotopic bladder reconstruction
    - cystectomy with continent urinary diversion
- Pre-operative radiotherapy with subsequent cystectomy

Primary radiotherapy. In the UK, radiotherapy is the most common first-line treatment offered to patients with invasive bladder cancer (Figure 7.3). Radiotherapy is given in a variety of ways, with changes in the fractionation (the way the total dose is divided up) designed to achieve maximum effect on the tumour while minimizing side-effects. Typically, treatment would be given during a series of out-patient visits over a 6-week period. The field covered by the radiation will include the bladder, prostate and pelvic lymph nodes. Of necessity, some radiation damage will also occur to neighbouring structures, in particular, the rectum, small bowel and the ureters.

Early side-effects of radiotherapy include skin, bowel and bladder sensitivity, nausea and tiredness. Late effects include reduction in bladder capacity, frequency of bowel movements with haematuria and rectal bleeding. Occasionally, these effects can be severe and may even require surgical intervention. With good planning, careful dosimetry and supervision of treatment to allow dose alteration if side-effects develop, radiotherapy is usually well tolerated.

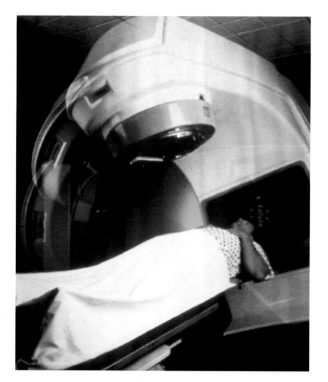

Figure 7.3
External-beam radiotherapy with a cobalt source for carcinoma of the bladder.

Radical surgery. In the USA and some European countries, patients are far more likely to be offered surgery as the initial treatment of their bladder tumour. The development of techniques avoiding ileal conduit diversion ('a bag') has helped to make surgery a more attractive option.

Cystectomy. The mainstay of surgical treatment of invasive bladder cancer is cystectomy involving removal of the bladder. As the whole of the urothelium has been exposed to whatever carcinogen initiated the cancer, the urethra must also be considered to be at risk of developing a tumour. For this reason, cystectomy is usually combined with total prostatectomy and urethrectomy (Figure 7.4). The urethra may be preserved, allowing construction of a new bladder from intestine, if there is no evidence of tumour in the prostatic urethra on biopsy and the bladder tumour is not associated with extensive CIS.

The operation is performed under general anaesthesia, using a trans-peritoneal approach. The lymph nodes draining the bladder are excised, the peritoneum over the bladder is divided and a plane between the bladder and

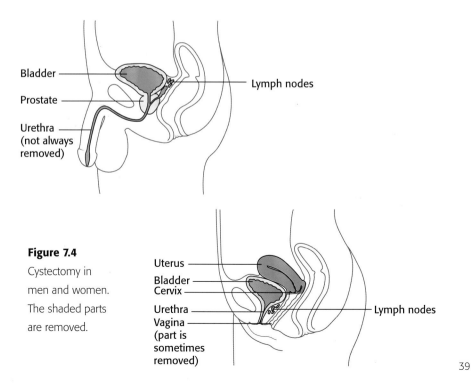

Figure 7.4

Cystectomy in men and women. The shaded parts are removed.

39

the rectum developed. The ureters are identified and divided, and the lateral pedicles of the bladder with its three main arteries ligated and divided. The prostate is mobilized, and if a new bladder is to be made, the urethra is divided at the base of the prostate. If a cystoprostatectomy and urethrectomy is being performed, the urethra is mobilized through a perineal incision and removed en bloc with the bladder and prostate.

The standard procedure offered to most patients involves isolating a loop of ileum attached to its vascular pedicle, anastomosing the ureters to one end of the loop and bringing the other end out of the abdominal wall as a stoma (an ileal conduit urinary diversion; Figure 7.5).

Orthotopic bladder reconstruction. It is possible to create a new bladder from intestinal segments using one of a variety of techniques. When this can be done without compromising the chance of cure, and when the patient is fit enough to withstand the extra surgery involved, the option of avoiding a urostomy is very attractive to the patient.

If a neobladder is to be fashioned, the dissection around the junction between the urethra and the prostate needs to be conducted with great care to preserve the distal sphincter. The new bladder can be made in a variety of

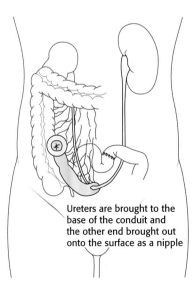

Ureters are brought to the base of the conduit and the other end brought out onto the surface as a nipple

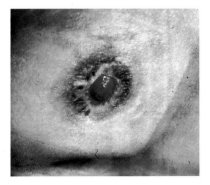

Figure 7.5 Patient with an ileal conduit urinary diversion.

ways, using small bowel, the ileocaecal segment or large bowel. The bowel is isolated on its vascular pedicle, opened along the antimesenteric border and sutured to create a pouch with a capacity of 400–800 ml (Figure 7.6). The ureters are anastomosed to the posterosuperior aspect of the pouch and an anastomosis performed between the most dependent part of the pouch and the urethral stump. This procedure takes longer than a standard cystectomy, and involves a longer hospital stay. It can be offered to women as well as men, despite earlier concerns about continence.

Creation of a continent stoma. In patients who are very keen to avoid a stoma draining into a bag, but in whom orthotopic reconstruction is not feasible (e.g. due to the presence of extensive CIS), a pouch can be made as described above. It is then brought to the surface using a continent, catheterizable stoma (Figure 7.7). The catheterizable stoma can be constructed from the appendix, tunnelled into the wall of the pouch so as

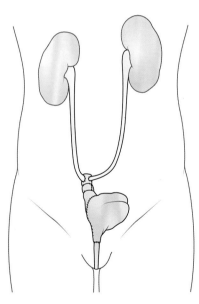

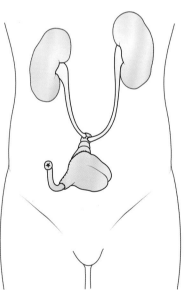

Figure 7.6 A neobladder allows the patient to pass urine as normal during the day, though leakage may occur at night.

Figure 7.7 With a continent stoma, urine is drained using a catheter passed through the stoma and into the pouch.

to create a flap-valve effect. This allows passage of a catheter to empty the pouch periodically, while maintaining continence between emptyings.

Pre-operative radiotherapy and planned cystectomy. In order to minimize local recurrences after cystectomy in patients with deeply invasive tumours, a reduced dose of radiotherapy (around 40 Gray) may be given, followed a few weeks later by cystectomy. A large UK study of this technique in patients with T3 tumours failed to show any benefit, and this combination is now rarely used.

Salvage cystectomy when recurrent tumour is found in the bladder after full-dose radiotherapy is still widely practised in the UK. If re-staging at the time of tumour recurrence shows no evidence of metastatic spread, these patients may still be cured of their disease.

Treatment outcomes

The results of radiotherapy or surgery depend on the grade and stage of the tumour. Overall 5-year survival rates following cystectomy are:
- pT2 disease: 60–80%
- pT3a disease: 50–70%
- pT3b disease: 30–60%.

Approximately 50% of all patients undergoing 'curative' treatment for bladder cancer will develop metastatic disease and die within 2 years of treatment.

Survival rates with radiotherapy are probably similar to those of surgery, but as exact pathological staging of the tumour and lymph nodes cannot be performed, direct comparisons are difficult. About 50% of patients undergoing radiotherapy will develop tumour recurrence in their bladder, and if there is no evidence of metastatic disease, may undergo salvage cystectomy.

In many parts of Europe and in the USA, cystectomy and reconstruction is the preferred treatment option for invasive bladder cancer. As this option becomes more widely available in the UK, there may be a move from radiotherapy to surgery as a primary treatment.

Quality of life following surgery for invasive bladder cancer

The prime concern of most patients with bladder cancer is to be cured of the disease. Apart from concerns about mortality, symptoms such as severe frequency, dysuria, urgency, haematuria and bladder pain may be sufficient to justify cystectomy even if cure is not possible. Relief of these symptoms represents a great improvement in a patient's quality of life.

The negative effects of cystectomy must be carefully explained to patients prior to embarking on surgery. In men, ejaculation will not occur, and those in whom erections are maintained will experience altered sensation at orgasm. Erectile failure is likely, even if attempts are made to spare the nerve supply to the corpora cavernosa, which passes close to the prostate; 70–100% of men will be impotent after cystectomy. In women, a conventional cystectomy includes hysterectomy and excision of the anterior vaginal wall, which will narrow the vagina and may cause dyspareunia. The operation can be modified in sexually active women to preserve vaginal volume. The patient must learn to cope with a urostomy, unless a bladder reconstruction or a continent diversion has been constructed.

While orthotopic bladder reconstruction eliminates the need for a stoma, the new bladder does not function like a normal one, and brings problems of its own, such as incontinence. With careful attention to technique, diurnal continence rates of 85% have been achieved. Most patients who experience problems do so at night, and a condom drainage system may be used. Another problem experienced is inadequate emptying. Most patients learn how to empty their bladder by relaxing the sphincter and increasing intra-abdominal pressure. If this does not achieve satisfactory results, intermittent self-catheterization may be necessary. A continent urinary diversion suffers from the same problems as a neobladder, except that difficulties with the catheterizable stoma replace problems with the sphincter mechanism. As the bowel segment secretes mucus, and as emptying may not always be complete, UTIs are likely to occur. Providing the ureters have been implanted with an anti-reflux technique, ascending infection should not be a problem.

In spite of the many potential difficulties with continent diversions or orthotopic bladder replacement, they offer a significant psychological benefit to patients undergoing cystectomy.

CHAPTER 8

Management of advanced disease

Patients with tumour extending outside the limits treated by radiotherapy or removed surgically have a very poor prognosis. Only 10% of patients with T4 disease will survive 5 years, and of those with known metastatic tumour, 95% will die within a year. The management of these patients must be directed to improving quality of life rather than longevity. Symptoms that may require palliation can be local or distant.

Local symptoms

Irritative voiding symptoms, such as urgency, frequency, dysuria and strangury, can cause extreme discomfort. Haematuria may be sufficient to require regular blood transfusions and may even be life-threatening. Clot retention of urine may require repeated visits to the hospital for emergency treatment.

Distant symptoms

Bone pain from metastases may be severe and distressing in its own right. Even more suffering may be caused if the metastasis involves a long bone and pathological fracture ensues. Cord compression from vertebral collapse or rapidly expanding dural deposits is one of the most severe symptoms a patient has to endure. Once established, there is little chance of recovery of motor or sensory function and the patient is likely to end his/her life in a wheelchair, incontinent of urine and faeces. For this reason, any symptoms suggesting early cord compression (paraesthesia in the legs, loss of power, or loss of bladder or bowel control) in a patient with malignant disease must be treated as a medical emergency. Immediate treatment with dexamethasone, followed by surgical decompression or radiotherapy may prevent progression to paraplegia.

Uraemia, characterized by anorexia, malaise, an unpleasant taste in the mouth and occasionally oliguria, may be due to ureteric obstruction. The decision to treat or not to treat renal failure in the presence of incurable malignancy is not an easy one. Renal failure may present a relatively rapid and pain-free escape from a terminal illness. Alternatively, a patient who is otherwise fairly asymptomatic may request relief of the obstruction. Careful explanation of the pros and cons of this decision to the patient and his/her relatives is required.

Other systemic symptoms, such as a cough from pulmonary deposits, malignant pleural effusion, capsular pain or jaundice from liver metastases and anaemia due to bone marrow replacement, are all common in advanced metastatic bladder cancer.

Whatever treatment is planned, the patient and their next of kin should be fully involved in the decision-making process. It must be made clear that the aim of treatment is palliation and not cure, and full explanation given of what can be expected.

Control of local symptoms

It is always worth excluding a UTI, which patients with necrotic tumours are more likely to develop. Treatment may reduce irritative symptoms, but haematuria can be very difficult to treat. Possible treatments are outlined in Table 8.1. Alum can be administered over 24–48 hours as a 5% solution via a three-way irrigating catheter. It is non-toxic and has little, if any, effect on bladder capacity. Formalin is more effective at stopping bleeding, but is more hazardous. It is used as a 4% solution, instilled into the bladder for 15 minutes and then drained via a catheter. The procedure must be done under general anaesthetic as it is very painful. Following treatment, the bladder capacity may be drastically reduced causing severe frequency or incontinence; reflux into the kidneys may cause renal failure. Palliative cystectomy may be justified in a reasonably fit patient with minimal

---

TABLE 8.1

Treatment of haematuria in metastatic bladder cancer

- Transurethral resection and fulguration: if tumour still present
- Palliative irradiation of the bladder: if radiotherapy not used previously; median survival 5–12 months following treatment
- Irrigation with alum or formalin solution: if earlier irradiation unsuccessful
- Palliative cystectomy: for patients with intractable bleeding or intolerable irritative symptoms

metastatic disease. In practice, few patients qualify for major surgery and the median survival for those who do is less than 12 months.

Control of distant symptoms

Bone pain can be controlled initially with non-steroidal anti-inflammatory drugs, but the possibility of pathological fractures must be borne in mind, especially if the spine or long bones are involved. Radiotherapy is very effective in relieving bone pain and is usually given to the affected area in one or two fractions. If multiple bones are involved (Figure 8.1), strontium-90 (metastron) may be given intravenously as a single bolus dose. It is taken up selectively by areas of increased bone turnover, thereby irradiating the metastatic deposits in the skeleton. Radiotherapy may also be given to soft tissue deposits if they are causing pain or threatening compression of vital structures.

Transfusion may be needed if anaemia causes symptoms, although the benefit is short-lived and repeated transfusions may be necessary. If the anaemia is due to iron deficiency from continuing haematuria, iron supplements are indicated. Often the anaemia is due to marrow replacement by tumour, and supplements are contraindicated.

The question of whether to treat obstructive renal failure in advanced malignancy is a difficult one. Usually, if the tumour has not yet been treated with the best available therapy, then nephrostomy drainage or internal ureteric stenting is appropriate. In patients whose tumour has advanced in spite of treatment, it is often kinder to withhold treatment and allow the patient to die peacefully.

The role of chemotherapy in palliation of advanced bladder cancer is limited. The toxicity of the drugs is compounded by renal impairment and general debility. Even when chemotherapy is given in full dosage, complete response (disappearance of all measurable deposits) is rare (about 20% in most studies) and response duration is only 10–18 months on average. The most effective regimen in use is M-VAC (methotrexate, vinblastine, adriamycin and cisplatinum).

Pain relief

When the treatments listed above are no longer controlling pain, specialist input from a palliative care team should be enlisted. All centres treating

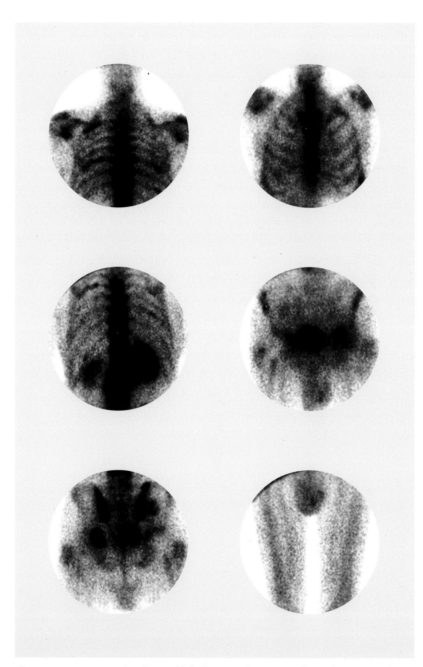

Figure 8.1 Bone scan showing multiple 'hot spots' corresponding to bony secondary deposits from carcinoma of the bladder.

patients with malignant disease should have strong links with such a team, and local guidelines should exist for the stage at which patients should be referred. There is much to be said for the early introduction of palliative care specialists. They have special skills in helping patients come to terms with the knowledge that their life expectancy is limited. Even if no direct intervention is needed following the first meeting, it will reassure the patient to know that they are available, and will inspire confidence when the time comes to call on their services. This support can often allow the patient to stay in their own home during most or all of their terminal illness. The palliative care team will work closely with the patient's family physician to achieve this.

In addition to the optimum use of opiate analgesics, the palliative care team may be able to offer nerve blocks, epidural injections, trans-epidermal nerve stimulation or acupuncture to provide pain relief. Other troublesome symptoms such as nausea, itching, dyspnoea and depression can often be helped by appropriate drug therapy. Sadly, in spite of the best efforts of surgeons and radiotherapists, the majority of patients with invasive bladder cancer will die of their disease. It is important that the doctors caring for these patients are aware of how much impact the quality of life has, not just on the patient, but on relatives and friends as well.

CHAPTER 9
Future trends

The mortality and morbidity of bladder cancer could be reduced by:
- disease prevention
- earlier diagnosis
- improvements in existing treatments
- development of new treatments.

Prevention

A number of bladder carcinogens have now been identified. The recognition of the carcinogenic properties of aniline dyes and aromatic amines used in industrial processes has led to them being banned. The most common carcinogen involved in bladder cancer – cigarette smoke – has escaped such a fate. Smoking is probably responsible for 30–40% of bladder cancer, and the association between bladder cancer and smoking is stronger than that for lung cancer. In patients with superficial tumours, the recurrence rate is higher and the chance of progression to invasive disease is higher in those who continue to smoke. It follows that the single greatest preventive measure would be to eliminate cigarette smoking. As this is politically unacceptable, we must continue to inform the public of the health hazards of this practice.

One of the more common causes of bladder cancer worldwide is infection with *Schistosoma haematobium*. Public health measures to eliminate schistosomiasis have been hindered in some countries by economic difficulties and political uncertainty.

Apart from the avoidance of known carcinogens, there is little else that can be done to prevent bladder cancer at present.

Earlier diagnosis

Screening. The increased use of urine dipstick testing for haematuria may lead to detection of some tumours at an earlier stage. Populations at high risk because of industrial exposure are routinely screened by this method. Voided urine cytology is not sufficiently sensitive to be used for routine screening. Some of the new antigen tests, such as Bard's BTA *stat* assay, may prove to have a role in diagnosis, but are too expensive for mass screening and will probably be more useful in the follow up of patients with known tumours.

Prompt presentation. All too often, patients with bladder tumours experience considerable delay in diagnosis. This may be because the patient does not report an isolated episode of haematuria, because the primary care physician ignores non-persistent haematuria, or because of delays imposed by the healthcare system.

It is vital that patients and their primary care physicians are aware that bleeding from a bladder tumour may be intermittent, and that a single episode of haematuria must be investigated. The process of hospital referral can be accelerated by establishing one-stop haematuria clinics.

Improvements in existing treatments

Advances have been made recently in defining the risk that patients with superficial disease face of local recurrence and progression to invasive disease. By considering factors such as tumour grade, number of tumours at presentation, presence of associated CIS and pattern of recurrence, patients can be divided into low-, intermediate- and high-risk groups. This allows a reduction in the frequency of cystoscopies in the low-risk group, and early introduction of intravesical chemotherapy with closer follow-up of those at greater risk. Recognition of the life-threatening behaviour of extensive CIS and grade 3 T1 tumours has brought about a more aggressive treatment policy, with early radical surgery being offered if intravesical BCG or mitomycin C fail to eradicate the tumour.

Additional information about the potential for progression in patients with superficial disease may be available by studying *p53* expression. This gene codes for a tumour suppressor and *p53* mutation is associated with an increased risk of invasion; thus, expression levels may identify those patients needing BCG or early cystectomy.

Earlier recourse to cystectomy or radiotherapy in patients with muscle-invasive disease should improve survival, and patient and surgeon reluctance to consider radical treatment will be reduced by the availability of techniques that avoid a urostomy. Unfortunately, adjuvant chemotherapy in patients undergoing surgery has not improved survival significantly.

Development of new treatments

The search for effective systemic cytotoxic therapy continues, with new drugs and drug combinations being evaluated. If chemotherapy can achieve a significant complete response rate in advanced disease, the hope of effective adjuvant therapy in early disease might be realized.

Improvements in the response of superficial disease through the use of drugs to counter tumour resistance to intravesical chemotherapy show promise, but have yet to be evaluated in a clinical setting. The treatment of superficial disease using photodynamic therapy is being explored. Certain drugs, given either systemically or intravesically, are taken up by the tumour cells. When exposed to light of a specific wave length from a laser, the drugs have a cytotoxic effect on the tumour cells. Clinical trials of this form of therapy are at an early stage. The evaluation of genetic markers of the potential for invasion may help define those patients with superficial disease at most risk of progression, who would benefit from more aggressive treatment.

At present, there seems little possibility of preventing bladder cancer, and curing metastatic disease remains a distant prospect. The best chances of minimizing the ravages of this disease will be gained by ensuring prompt diagnosis, and then targeting high-risk patients with the most appropriate therapy at an early stage. We hope that, in a small way, *Fast Facts – Bladder Cancer* can help towards meeting these objectives.

Key references

EPIDEMIOLOGY AND AETIOLOGY

Bostwick DG. Natural history of early bladder cancer. *J Cell Biol* 1992;161 (Suppl):31–8.

Dalbagni G, Presti J, Reuter V, Fair WR, Cordon Cardo C. Genetic alterations in bladder cancer. *Lancet* 1993;342:469–71.

Morrison AS, Buring JE, Verhoek WG *et al.* An international study of smoking and bladder cancer. *J Urol* 1984;131:650–4.

Parker SL, Tong T, Bolden S, Wingo PA. Cancer Statistics, 1997. *CA Cancer J Clin* 1997;47:5–27.

Thompson IM, Peek M, Rodriguez FR. The impact of cigarette smoking on stage, grade and number of recurrences in transitional cell carcinoma of the bladder. *J Urol* 1987;137:401–3.

Vineis P. The use of biomarkers in epidemiology: the example of bladder cancer. *Toxicol Lett* 1992;463:64–5.

Wolf H, Melsen F, Pedersen SE, Nielsen KT. Natural history of carcinoma in situ of the urinary bladder. *Scan J Urol Nephrol* 1994;157(Suppl):147–51.

PATHOLOGY

Addis T. The number of formed elements in the urinary sediment of normal individuals. *J Clin Invest* 1926;2:409–15.

Presti JC Jr, Reuter VE, Galan T, Fair WR, Cordon Cardo C. Molecular genetic alterations in superficial and locally advanced human bladder cancer. *Cancer Res* 1991;51:5405–9.

Sandberg AA, Berger CS. Review of chromosome studies urological tumors. II. Cytogenetics and molecular genetics of bladder cancer. *J Urol* 1994;151:545–60.

CLINICAL PRESENTATION OF THE BLADDER

Hastie KJ, Hamdy FC, Collins MC, Williams JL. Upper tract tumours following cystectomy for bladder cancer. Is routine intravenous urography worthwhile? *Br J Urol* 1991;67:29–31.

Lynch T, Waymont J, Dunn M *et al.* Repeat testing for haematuria and underlying urological pathology. *Br J Urol* 1994;74:730–2.

Mommsen S, Aargard J, Sell A. Presenting symptoms, treatment delay and survival in bladder cancer. *Scand J Urol Nephrol* 1983;17:163–7.

INVESTIGATIONS

Mufti GR, Singh M. Value of random mucosal biopsies in the management of superficial bladder cancer. *Eur Urol* 1992;22:288–93.

Palou J, Farina LA, Villavicencio H, Vicente J. Upper tract urothelial tumor after transurethral resection for bladder tumor. *Eur Urol* 1992;21:110–14.

Witjes JA, Kiemeney LALM, Verbeek ALM, Heijbroek RP, Debruyne FMJ, and members of the Dutch South East Cooperative Urological Group. Random bladder biopsies and the risk of recurrent superficial bladder cancer: a prospective study in 126 patients. *World J Urol* 1992;10:231–4.

MICROSCOPIC HAEMATURIA

Frennis S, Heedrick G, Holt C *et al.* Centrifugation techniques and reagent strips in the assessment of microhaematuria. *J Clin Pathol* 1977;30:336–40.

Yasuma T, Koikawa Y, Uozumi J *et al.* Clinical study of asymptomatic microscopic haematuria. *Int J Urol Nephrol* 1994;26:1–6.

MANAGEMENT OF SUPERFICIAL DISEASE

Bouffioux C, Kurth KH, Bono A *et al.* Intravesical adjuvant chemotherapy for superficial transitional cell bladder carcinoma: Results of two European Organization for Research and Treatment of Cancer randomized trials with mitomycin C and doxorubicin comparing early versus delayed instillations and short-term versus long-term treatment. *J Urol* 1996;153:934–41.

Cookson MS, Sarosdy MF. Management of stage T1 superficial bladder cancer with intravesical BCG therapy. *J Urol* 1992; 148:797–801.

Fitzpatrick JM. The natural history of superficial bladder carcinoma. *Semin Urol* 1993;11:127–36.

Fradet Y, Tardif M, Bourget L, Robert J. Clinical cancer progression in urinary bladder tumours evaluated by multiparameter flow cytometry with monoclonal antibodies. Laval University Urology Group. *Cancer Res* 1990;50: 432–7.

Glashan RW. A randomized control study of intravesical alpha-2b-interferon in carcinoma in situ of the bladder. *J Urol* 1990;144:658–61.

Heney NM. Natural history of superficial bladder cancer. Prognostic features and long-term disease course. *Urol Clin North Am* 1992;19:429–33.

Herr HW, Wartinger DD, Fair WR, Oettgen HF. Bacillus Calmette-Guérin therapy for superficial bladder cancer: a 10-year follow-up. *J Urol* 1992;147: 1020–3.

Hudson MA *et al.* p53 protein accumulation in superficial bladder cancer is a predictor of subsequent muscle invasion. *J Urol Pathol* 1994;2:307–18.

Jaske G and members of the EORTC-GU Group. Intravesical instillation of BCG in carcinoma in situ of the urinary bladder. In: Debruyne FMJ, Denis L, van der Meijden APM, eds. *BCG in Superficial Bladder Cancer: Proceedings of an EORTC Genitourinary Group Meeting.* New York: Alan R Liss, 1989:187–92.

Kurth KH, Schroeder FH, Tunn U *et al.* Adjuvant chemotherapy of superficial transitional cell bladder carcinoma: preliminary results of a European Organization for Research on Treatment of Cancer randomized trial comparing doxorubicin hydrochloride, ethoglucid and transurethral resection alone. *J Urol* 1984;132:258–62.

Lamm DL, Blumenstein BA, Crawford ED et al. A randomized trial of intravesical doxorubicin and immunotherapy with bacille Calmette-Guérin for transitional cell carcinoma of the bladder. N Engl J Med 1991;325:1205–9.

Lamm DL. Complications of bacillus Calmette-Guérin immunotherapy. Urol Clin North Am 1992;19:565–72.

Malkowicz SB, Skinner DG. Development of upper tract carcinoma after cystectomy for bladder cancer. Urology 1990;36:20–2.

Morales A, Eidinger D, Bruce AW. Adjuvant immunotherapy with BCG in recurrent superficial bladder cancer. In: Lamoureux G et al., eds. BCG in Cancer Immunotherapy. New York; Grune & Stratton, 1976:247–52.

Nadler RB, Catalona WJ, Hudson MA, Ratliff TL. Durability of the tumor-free response for intravesical bacillus Calmette-Guérin therapy. J Urol 1994;152:367–73.

Newling D. Intravesical therapy in the management of superficial transitional cell carcinoma of the bladder: the experience of the EORTC group. Br J Cancer 1990;61:497–9.

Okamura T, Tozawa K, Yamada Y, Sakagami H, Ueda K, Kohri K. Clinicopathological evaluation of repeated courses of intravesical bacillus Calmette-Guérin instillation for preventing recurrence of initially resistant superficial bladder cancer. J Urol 1996;156:967–71.

Pagano F, Garbeglio A, Milani C, Bassi P, Pegoraro V. Prognosis of bladder cancer. I. Risk factors in superficial transitional cell carcinoma. Eur Urol 1987;13:145–9.

Sarosdy MF, Hudson MA, Ellis WJ et al. Improved detection of recurrent bladder cancer using the BARD BTA stat Test. Urology 1997;50:349–53.

Sarosdy MF, deVere White RW, Soloway MS et al. Results of a multicenter trial using the BTA test to monitor for and diagnose recurrent bladder cancer. J Urol 1995;154:379–83.

Sarosdy MF. Principles of intravesical chemotherapy and immunotherapy. Urol Clin North Am 1992;19:509–19.

Sarosdy MF, Lamm D, Williams R et al. Phase 1 trial of oral bropirimine in superficial bladder cancer. J Urol 1992;147:31–3.

Sarosdy MF, Lowe BA, Schellhammer PF et al. Oral bropirimine immunotherapy of carcinoma in situ of the bladder: Results of a phase II trial. Urology 1996;48:21–7.

Schmeller NT, Hofstetter AG. Laser treatment of ureteral tumors. J Urol 1989;141:840–3.

Soloway MS, Briggman JV, Carpinito GA et al. Use of a new tumour marker, urinary NMP-22, in the detection of occult or rapidly recurring transitional cell carcinoma of the urinary tract following surgical treatment. J Urol 1996;156: 363–7.

Vegt PDJ, Witjes JA, Witjes WPJ, Doesburg WH, Debruyne FM, van der Meijden AP. A randomized study of intravesical mitomycin C, bacillus Calmette-Guérin Tice and bacillus Calmette-Guérin RIVM treatment in pTa-pT1 papillary carcinoma and carcinoma in situ of the bladder. J Urol 1995;153:929–33.

MANAGEMENT OF MUSCLE-INVASIVE DISEASE

Bloom H, Hendry W, Wallace D *et al.*
Treatment of T3 bladder cancer:
controlled trial of preoperative
radiotherapy and radical cystectomy
versus radical radiotherapy. Second report
and review. *Br J Urol* 1982;54:136–42.

Fossa S, Woehre H, Aass N *et al.*
Definitive radiation therapy of muscle
invasive bladder cancer: a retrospective
review of 317 patients. *Cancer*
1993;72:3036–45.

Skinner D, Lieskowsky G. Management
of invasive and high grade bladder cancer.
In: *Diagnosis and Management of
Genitourinary Cancer.* Philadelphia:
Saunders, 1988:1–295.

MANAGEMENT OF ADVANCED DISEASE

Schwartz CB, Bekirov H, Melman A.
Urothelial tumors of upper tract following
treatment of primary bladder transitional
cell carcinoma. *Urology* 1992;40:509–11.

Sternberg CN, Yagoda A, Scher HI.
M-VAC for advanced transitional cell
carcinoma of the urothelium: efficacy and
patterns of response and relapse. *Cancer*
1989;64:2448–58.

Index

see also microscopic
haematuria
high-powered field (HPF) 4, 24
histology 8–10, 21, 28–9
history-taking 19

adenocarcinoma 8, 10, 13
adjuvant therapy 10, 12
advanced disease 44–8
distant symptoms 44–5
control 46
local symptoms 44
control 45–6
pain relief 46, 48
aetiology 5–7
anaplasia 4, 8, 12
anorexia 16, 44
atypia 10, 29

bacillus Calmette-Guérin (BCG)
immunotherapy 4, 12, 30–2,
33, 50
complications 32
bacterial cystitis 14
biopsy 22–3, 29
bladder reconstruction 40–2
bladder tumour antigen (BTA)
test 4, 19, 34
bone pain 44, 46

carcinoma in situ (CIS) 4, 8, 10,
11, 12, 15, 21, 22, 30, 31, 33,
39, 41, 50
chemotherapy 30–2, 46, 50, 51
clinical presentation 14–18
computed tomography (CT) 4,
20, 35, 36
cystectomy 4, 10, 12, 30, 33, 35,
37, 39–40, 41, 42–3, 45, 50
cystoscopy 4, 18, 20–1, 29, 33,
34, 35, 50
cytology 21, 33, 34

diagnosis 26–7
delayed 15, 17–18, 50
dysplasia 4, 10, 11, 21, 29
dysuria 14, 15, 42

elderly people 5
epidemiology 5

genetic changes 7
genetic markers 51
grading 10, 12

haematuria 14, 15, 19, 42,
44, 45

impotence 43
incidence 5
industrial exposure 6, 49
indwelling catheters 7,8
intravenous urogram (IVU)
4, 16, 18, 19, 20
intravesical immunotherapy
4, 12, 30–2, 50
invasion through bladder
wall 11
investigations 19–23
irritative symptoms 14, 15,
44, 45

known bladder carcinogens 6

lymph node involvement 11,
12, 13
lymphadenopathy 35

magnetic resonance imaging
(MRI) 4, 20, 36, 37
male:female ratio 5
metabolic complications 16
metastases 11, 12, 13, 17, 35,
36, 44, 45, 51
microscopic haematuria 15,
24–7
mortality 12–13
muscle-invasive disease 12,
35–43
staging 35–6
treatment options 36–42
outcomes 42–3

nuclear matrix protein (NMP)
test 4, 19, 34

pain 14, 16, 44, 46
relief 46, 48
palliative care team 46, 48
pathology 8–13, 14, 21
patterns of recurrence and
spread 10–12
photodynamic therapy 51
physical examination 19
primary CIS 4, 8
prognosis 8, 10, 12–13, 44
progression 10, 11, 12, 51

proteinuria 25, 26

quality of life 42–3, 48

radiotherapy
as cause 7
as treatment 35, 37, 38, 42,
45, 46, 50
side-effects 38
recurrence 6, 10, 12, 50
surveillance 33–4
renal failure 44, 45, 46
risk factors 5–7
chromosomal changes 7
chronic infection 7, 8
cigarette smoking 5–6, 49
dietary factors 6
drugs 6–7
occupational 6
radiation 7

schistosomiasis 7, 8, 49
secondary CIS 4, 8
smoking as prime cause 5–6, 49
squamous cell carcinoma 8, 13
staging 35–6
see also TNM staging
stoma 41–2, 43
superficial disease 28–34
intravesical therapy 30–2
prognostic factors 28–9
prognostic groups 29–30
surveillance 33–4
surgery 12, 21–2, 28, 35
radical 37, 39–42
survival rates 42
symptoms 14–18
systemic 14, 15, 16

TNM staging 4, 10, 11
transitional cell carcinoma
(TCC) 4, 8, 9, 12, 26
transurethral resection 21–2,
28, 35
treatment delay 18
tumour markers 34

ultrasonography 20
undifferentiated carcinomas 10
urinalysis 15, 19, 24–5
urinary tract infection (UTI)
4, 45
recurrent 14, 15, 16
urine cytology 18
urography 4